Qua

MW00364593

Quartz Crystals

A guide to identifying quartz crystals
and their healing properties

Isabel Silveira

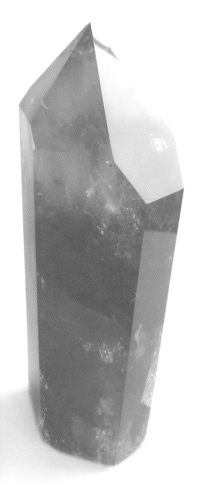

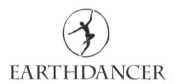

EARTHDANCER

A FINDHORN PRESS IMPRINT

Publisher's note

The information in this volume has been compiled according to the best of our knowledge and belief, and the healing properties of the crystals have been tested many times over. Bearing in mind that different people react in different ways, neither the publisher nor the author can give a guarantee as to the effectiveness or safety of use in individual cases. In the case of serious health problems please consult your doctor or naturopath.

Quartz Crystals:
A guide to identifying quartz crystals and their healing properties
Isabel Silveira

First edition 2008

This English edition © 2008 Earthdancer GmbH
English translation © 2008 Gisele Aparecida Cossas Farias Brierley
Editing of the translated text by Claudine Bloomfield

Originally published in Portuguese as *Ampliando nossa visão do Reino Mineral*

World Copyright © Totalidade Editora, São Paulo, 2007
Original Portuguese text copyright © Isabel Silveira 2007

All rights reserved. No part of this book may be reprinted or reproduced or utilised in any form or by any electronic, mechanical, or other means, now known or hereafter invented, including photo-copying and recording, or in any information storage or retrieval system, without permission in writing from the publisher.

Cover Photography: Manfred Feig
Cover Design: Dragon Design, GB
Photos: Manfred Feig
Typesetting and graphics: Dragon Design UK
Typeset in Hiroshige and Rotis Sans Serif
Printed and bound in China

ISBN 978-0-84409-148-5

Published by Earthdancer, an imprint of:
Findhorn Press, 305a The Park, Forres IV36 3TE, Scotland.
www.earthdancerbooks.com, www.findhornpress.com

Gratitude, reverence and love to the Great Goddess

and also

to Mother Earth;

to the Stone People;

to Ilse Whately Simões (in memoriam) and Beatriz Simões do Amaral who, even without knowing it, sowed the seed of who I am today;

to Antonio Duncan (in memoriam), my eternal Crystal master;

to Mano and Cláudia from Espaço Zym, for the trust both placed in me, and for the opportunity of having a space in which I could share my Crystal experiences;

to all my students, especially Manfred and Sílvia, who were responsible for this book.

Contents

PREFACE

Dear reader,

This small book came into existence through the efforts of my students, especially Manfred Feig and Sílvia Guerra. Imagine what it is like for me, someone without a degree in literature, to see my efforts crowned in this way. I am very happy!

My students immediately recognized that which I hoped to achieve with this book - to present information about crystals in an objective, concise, and yet profound way.

My purpose was to allow you, the reader, to accurately and quickly identify different forms of quartz and uncover the energetic properties of each piece.

All the information gathered in this book is the result of my studies - especially those undertaken with my master Antonio Duncan - and of my own experiences with the Mineral Realm. An example is the name 'aggregator', which is a name I was inspired to create for the crystal usually called 'barnacle'; the name came to me during my own learning process with that particular crystal.

Crystals 'speak' to the soul of each one of us in a unique and exclusive way. They 'call us', attract us, in a way that is always in tune with the moment we are currently living and in accordance with our capacity to understand and process information, change and transformation.

Therefore, dear reader, you must expand upon all the information in this book. I believe there are no absolute truths, no rights or wrongs in any aspect of our existence, especially in our relationship to crystals. What exists is just what is good and truthful for us in a specific moment in our lives.

May the Infinite Light guide your steps in this Crystalline Journey.

Isabel
Spring 2007

INTRODUCTION

Archaeological excavations carried out all over the world have shown that mankind has always used precious stones, and somehow knew *how* to use them.

Progress and technology have brought back to our daily lives the power of these stones, a power that can no longer be denied. Crystals are now used in computer chips, scanners, and in an enormous variety of other electronic and high precision equipment.

Crystals are recognized as excellent energy conductors – the purest and the most accurate.

HOW CAN CRYSTALS HELP US?

A crystal is a tuner

A crystal works exactly like a radio dial – it eliminates interference and allows us to be once again in tune with our own frequency.

To do this, the crystal cleanses our inner energy flow and re-organizes components of our electromagnetic fields, reinstating balance and harmony. Crystals therefore promote realignment with our own inner light, and bring the possibility of harmony to any issue we may be working on.

A crystal is 'frozen' light

A crystal is a portal of light created from the cosmic dust of a universe in eternal expansion, its many facets reflecting the innumerable dimensions of life.

A crystal's composition is pure and harmonious, with all of its molecules vibrating at precisely the same frequency. Therefore its electromagnetic field reproduces the purity and harmony of its own essence, 'contaminating' all the electromagnetic fields in its surroundings, which might include the electromagnetic fields of a place, a human being, an animal or a plant.

A crystal works by its very existence, regardless of whether we believe in its power or not.

A crystal also acts because of its chromatic and chemical properties

Colours are light frequencies with different levels of vibration and they have a direct influence on human consciousness. Crystals can absorb, reflect and radiate different light frequencies and transfer them to the human consciousness and organism.

Crystals have this capacity because their chemical nature can also be found within the human body: calcium, magnesium, copper, fluorine, silicon, etc. This action is explained by the homeopathic principle: 'like cures like'.

THE
QUARTZ
FAMILY

Quartzes are among the most common minerals on our planet, and they appear in a great variety of types and colours.

This book focuses on a small grouping within this great family: white quartz (also known as clear quartz), citrine, amethyst, smoky, tangerine and rosy quartz. I have chosen these crystals because they appear in different forms through which they reveal their nature. I will be explaining this in the chapter - *The Crystals and their Forms*.

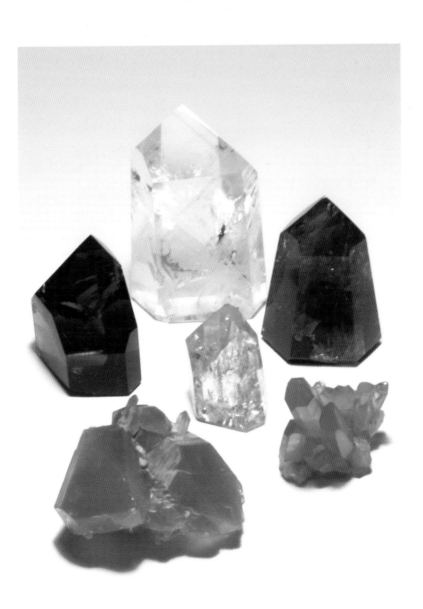

CLEAR QUARTZ

- Vibrates pure white light, which contains all the other colours.

- Represents a perfect material form, aligned and in harmony with cosmic forces.

- Referred to as 'solidified light'.

- Performs on all levels: physical, etheric, emotional, mental and spiritual.
  - Unblocks
  - Purifies
  - Balances
  - Activates
  - Amplifies
  - Protects

- Has the same effects upon a room or environment, and can be used to reduce and even eliminate the harmful effects of radiation.

Examples:

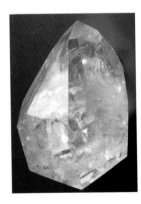 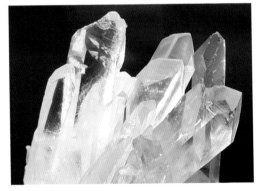

- A limpid quartz in shades of orange ranging from pale to intense.

- Channels and anchors pure creative energy in the material plane.
  - Works with all levels of creative energy, from the creativity that comes directly from the soul to the creativity it takes to resolve small day-to-day issues.

- Awakens and stimulates our creative expression on all levels.
  - Provides the clarity, focus and direction necessary for the practical application of creativity.

- Generates warmth, movement and joy.

Examples:

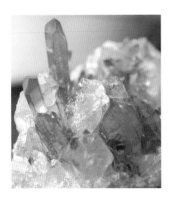
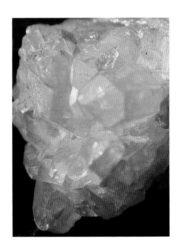

- Colour varies from the most intense lilac to a gentle lavender tone.

- The most common form is a druse.

- Difficult to find in nature with natural points (extremities), in rough or naturally polished forms.

- Amethysts with the special features and configurations detailed in this book are very rare.

- Especially indicated to teach us how to meditate:
  - Soothes thoughts, bringing tranquillity to the mind.
  - Encourages a shift in consciousness from constant mental activity to silence and inner peace.

- Transforms negative or unbalanced energies into peaceful and loving tranquillity.
  - Amethyst druses are excellent for use in communal rooms, such as the bathrooms, lobbies and waiting rooms of companies and clinics.

- Excellent for use during times of stress and tension, and can therefore help with the following:
  - Anxiety
  - Mood swings
  - Impatience and irritability
  - Insomnia
  - Agitated sleep or nightmares
  - Migraines and headaches

- On a more general physical level, amethyst can be used to treat:
  - The nervous system
  - Digestive disorders, such as gastritis and ulcerations

AMETHYST QUARTZ

amethyst

- Skin problems, especially acne
- Inflammation
- Fever

- Used since the Middle Ages in the treatment of alcoholism.

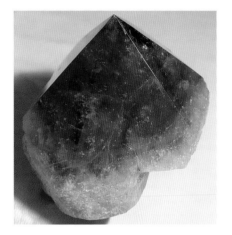

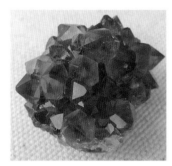

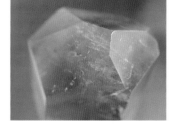

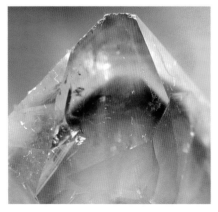

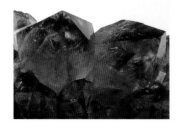

CITRINE QUARTZ

- Colours range from pale gold to golden brown.

- Manifests golden light in the physical plane.

- Like the sun, its energy gives warmth, comfort, power and life.

- Activates and amplifies our inner light, creating a positive and strong aura.

- Creates a vibrant force wherever and however it is used.

- Improves self esteem, correcting and balancing the sense of self.

- Stimulates activity in all the physical systems.

- Strengthens the physical and psychic bodies.

- Aids digestion and assimilation on both the physical and psychic levels.

- Activates one's inner light to help overcome the problems and challenges of everyday life. Excellent for people worn out by stress, a prolonged illness or a difficult emotional situation, and for those suffering from depression.

- Special tip: carry a citrine quartz with you when you need to overcome a negative emotional or mental state such as anger, jealousy, annoyance, insecurity, fear, powerlessness, a sense of failure, sadness, or ill-humour.

CITRINE QUARTZ

Examples:

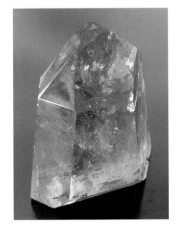
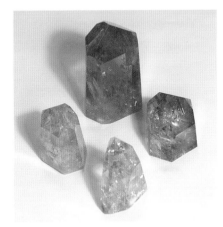

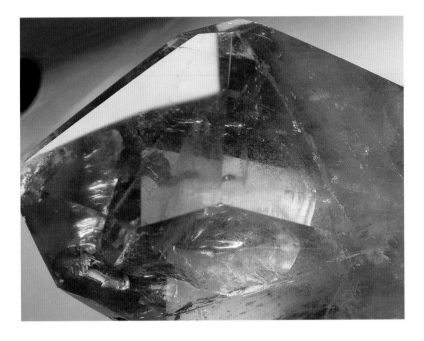

- Colour ranges from brown/grey to black, but is always transparent.

- Used to channel and anchor light in the material plane.

- Smoky quartz has dissolving and reconstructing properties:
  - Slowly, layer by layer, plane by plane, high-frequency vibrations dissolve deeply entrenched patterns that no longer serve us.
  - Then, starting from the base, a new structure is built, layer by layer, plane by plane.

- Encourages steadiness, stability and solidity.

- Acts upon issues relating to foundations, structure and accomplishment.

- Realigns our goals, making them objective and tangible.

- It supports our ability to relate to reality through really recognizing and understanding the circumstances in which we find ourselves, and through recognizing, accepting and working with our limitations:
  - Sinks roots into reality, deterring us from illusion or self delusion, and encouraging us to lay paths upon our own base.
  - An excellent 'protection shield', channelling and anchoring light in the physical plane.

- Improves our capacity to forge ahead, to build paths, and to break through.

- Helps us manifest the material conditions necessary for our stability.

SMOKY QUARTZ

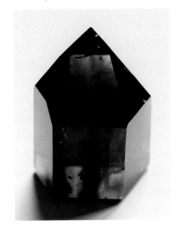

smoky quartz

Examples:

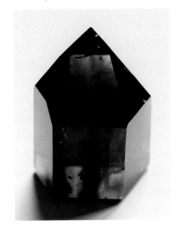

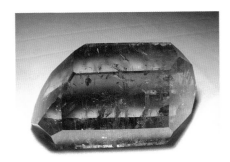

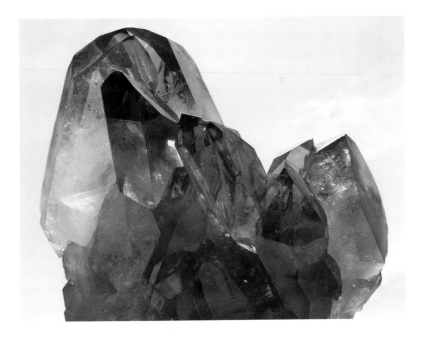

- Limpid pink-coloured quartz.

- Channels and anchors the pure energy of love in the physical plane.

- Awakens and stimulates our own energy of love.

- Gentle energy of comfort, calm, and shelter.

Examples:

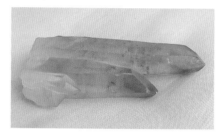

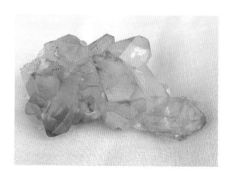

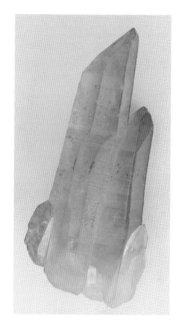

THE CRYSTALS AND THEIR FORMS

Most often, the term 'master crystals' is used to indicate only certain types of clear quartz crystals that present special features in their constitution or geometric configuration, some of which are are shown in this book: channelling and transmitter quartzes, window, Isis, laser, cathedral, twin and Dow. However, as a shamanic practitioner I have come to realise that everything is a teacher, and is part of Mother Earth's family. All that exists is sacred, a sacred extension of the Creator. Expressions such as 'Grandfather Sun', 'Stone People' and 'Standing People' (trees) indicate our respect for the sacred missions granted by the Great Mystery. Native peoples called this Medicine.

Considering all the above with great humility, I see ALL crystals and every being of the mineral realm as a 'master' or 'teacher', as every single one has a specific 'Medicine' that we can use to assist our development.

The combination of colour, features, geometric configuration, signs and textures open us to a universe of information and magic that combines with our personal sensations to allow a new vision and understanding of life. In shamanic language, this is *healing*.

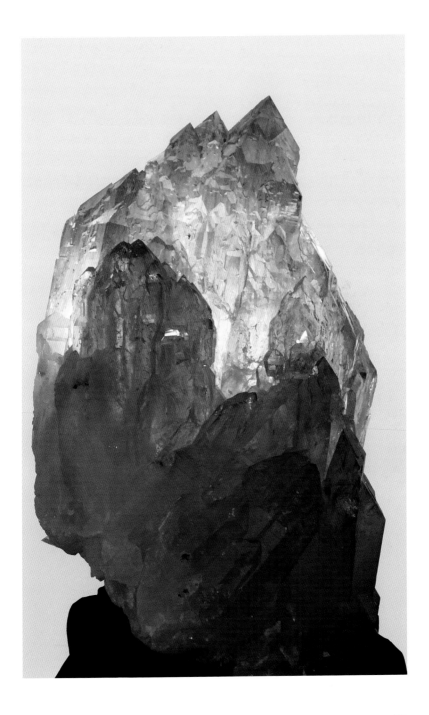

channelling quartz crystal

- A large, seven-sided face (heptagon) flanked by two small triangles, with another triangle directly behind it on the opposite side.

- Teaches us to appeal to our inner wisdom in order to recognize and channel our own inner light.

Example:

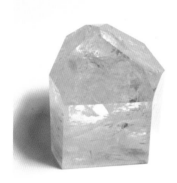 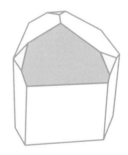

A crystal with a large, seven-sided face flanked by two small triangles, with another triangle directly behind it.

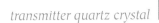
- A perfect triangle flanked by two seven-sided faces.

- Transmits human thought forms to the universal mind in order that they may be received and replied to.

- Main Function: Teaches us to 'ask and receive'.
  - It is of fundamental importance to be capable of expressing to the Universe that which we feel we need, and of receiving the answer when it is given.
  - Our thoughts create our physical reality: we have exactly what we have asked of the Universe.
  - If we don't have what we want, it's possible that we are not defining and transmitting what we want in a clear way, or that we are not capable of manifesting in our lives the effects of our thought projections (prayers).

Examples:

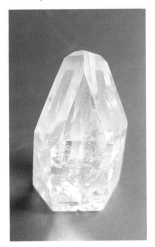

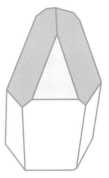

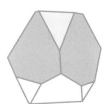

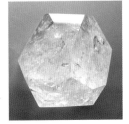

Three-sided face flanked by two seven-sided faces.

Bird's-eye view of a transmitter crystal.

29

WINDOW CRYSTAL

OR NATURALLY POLISHED CRYSTAL

window quartz crystal

- Identified by a lozenge cut into one of its sides.
  - The lozenge is natural, and is also called a 'diamond'.
  - Represents balance, integration and synthesis between soul/matter; above/below; inside/outside; superior/inferior.

- Takes us beyond all identities to the true Self, our divine essence.
  - Reflects the imperfections and shadows that stop us from expressing our divine essence, the Self.

- A *mirror*, clear and truthful, emitting back to the human consciousness exactly what is received.
  - *Does not retain* impressions or carry records.
  - Reflects only the person looking into it. Nothing of the person who used the crystal before will be seen or taken on.
  - We are reflected just as we are – the shadow and the light.

- A non-judgmental frame of mind is needed in order to work with this crystal; the window master crystal will reveal the aspect of ourselves that needs to be reviewed. To deal with what is reflected, we must free ourselves of thoughts, emotions, and any behaviour that blocks acceptance of the responsibility for living the truth. By 'truth' I mean the expression of the Self, or the divine essence in our lives.

- Increases its power as it continues to be used.

- Attracts and is attracted to those who need to look deeply within themselves.

- Relatively hard to find.

WINDOW CRYSTAL

OR NATURALLY POLISHED CRYSTAL

window quartz crystal

Examples:

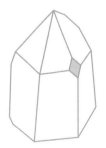

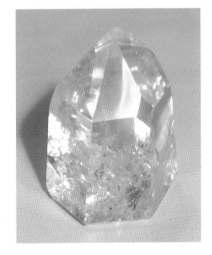

Window quartz crystal:

The drawing highlights the lozenge ('diamond') at the meeting point of four faces.

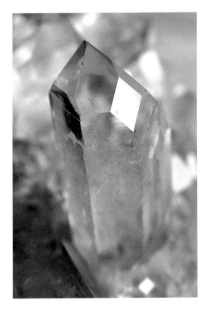

A window crystal in one point of a clear quartz druse.

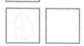

- Isis is a Goddess who was worshipped in Ancient Egypt. She personifies feminine power, the power of self-cure, inner strength, and the capacity to overcome the most lacerating of human grief – the violent and unjust death of a loved one. She represents determination, perseverance, and the power to renew life.

- An Isis crystal presents a face with the configuration of a pentagon (five-sided polygon). A horizontal base line connects with two other lines that go up, making angles slightly inclined to the outside. From these two short lines come two other, longer lines inclined to the inside that eventually unite at the top, completing the figure. The clearer the symmetry between the opposite sides, the more balanced (pure) the energy of the crystal.

- Represents the universal feminine principle; symbolizes the **Goddess**.

- Personifies the feminine power of creation that conceives and gives birth to all of creation.

- Activates and integrates the power of the **inner Goddess**.

- Isis represents:
  - The inexhaustible rebirth of all things
  - Determination
  - Perseverance
  - Life renewal
  - Victory of truth and justice
  - Determination and will power to win against evil
  - The courage to defend the truth
  - The courage to correct mistakes

ISIS CRYSTAL

- Inner power
- Ability to overcome obstacles

- An Isis crystal can be used:
  - In cases of depression.
  - When one has lost a loved one by death, mainly in cases of brutal death as a consequence of robbery, disaster, etc.
  - To cure the feeling of being wronged by life or by God.
  - When a serious illness is diagnosed, to help with the initial impact.
  - In cases where a person suffers financial loss, a job loss, or loss of 'status'.
  - When a person is suffering from some sort of injustice.

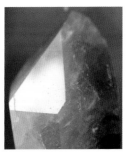

Various examples of the Isis crystal.

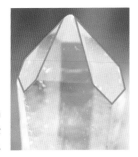

A rare example with two Isis faces in the same extremity.

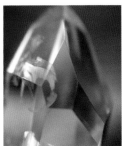

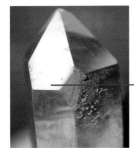

Face detail of an Isis crystal.

- Contains the secret of the laser.

- Origin: Stellar space. Laser crystals were transported to Earth and were used mainly in Lemurian temples of healing.
  - They carry the knowledge not only of ancient civilizations, but also of stellar space.
  - They often exhibit drawings or markings that are different from any other crystals and resemble hieroglyphs.
    - Marked lasers, specifically, have been used in Lemurian temples of healing.
    - The drawings and markings are records of the crystal's own experiences as it collected information about human conditions and how to heal them.
    - The more it has been used to heal, the more knowledge the crystal contains and the more depictions can be noted.

- Laser crystals often present a tabular form (like a bridge for union and integration with the Higher Self).

Some of the most common uses:

- To create power fields or protective shields around people and places:
  - In loco: surround the object, place or person, pointing crystals outwards.
  - With a mandala: In the centre of a mandala, place a symbol of that which needs protecting, surrounded by several lasers pointing outwards.

- Invisibility:
  - We do not actually disappear, but we project a light of such intensity around us that other people cannot see through it, thereby creating the illusion of disappearing.

laser quartz crystal

- A statement to reflect upon: *'The art of invisibility lies in the removal of attraction'.*

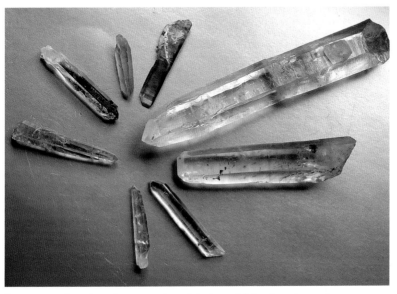

Laser crystal: various laser quartz points (wands) in clear, tangerine, citrine and smoky quartz. There are also rutilated pieces.

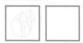

- Multiple points connected to the body of a main 'mother' crystal.

- There can be 'cathedrals' in clear, citrine and smoky quartz crystals.

- Cosmic computers that contain the 'Akashic records', a register of all known eras, to which all thoughts, words and actions of all living beings have been stored.
  - They are true 'libraries' that contain sacred universal knowledge, written in the language of light.
  - They register only those thought forms that are tuned to the Creator's Intelligence, the Supreme Universal Mind.
  - The work of this crystal is to convert such knowledge into a language that is intelligible to the human mind.

- For the individual, a cathedral quartz develops the concept of Sacred Space, a place inside ourselves where we can retreat in moments of meditation to seek our inner 'God', the divine spark in our hearts.

- In a larger sense, these crystals symbolize the 'Lord's dwelling', a place where God is recognized and revered (a cathedral), and also a place of knowledge and learning (a library).

Many examples of the cathedral quartz, with three or more terminations sharing the same body:

CATHEDRAL CRYSTAL

cathedral quartz crystal

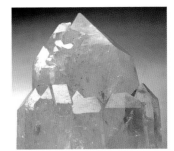

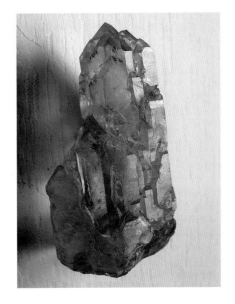

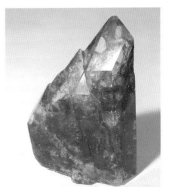

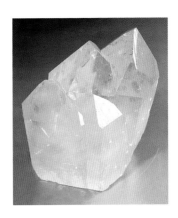

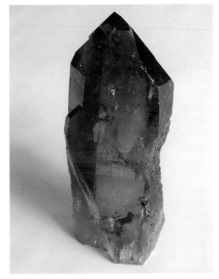

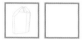

- Two points sharing the same main body.

- Contain the mysteries of divine connection with another being.

- The first great teaching of the twin crystal is the greatest union of all: the fusion of our soul with our inner Divine Essence.
  - This primary state of unity must be attained before unity with another.

- Once in tune with our own Divine Essence, we can recognize the Divine in others.
  - When this occurs we acquire a direct knowledge, transcending thoughts and words.

- We live in tune with our own essence and that of another.

- A twin crystal teaches us the secrets of soul partnership, and how it is possible to fuse with another being without losing one's own identity or personal power.

- Ultimately one can experience a state of unity with all people, beings and things:
  - Through absolute connection with the Divine Essence, we find unity with all other forms, all of which have originated from the same primordial source.

- A twin crystal that presents an Isis face at one of its terminations symbolizes the fusion of the soul with the universal feminine principle.

Please note
  - Generator: only one point.
  - Druse: two or more points sharing a common base.
  - Cathedral: three or more points sharing a single body.

TWIN CRYSTAL

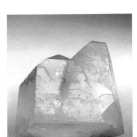
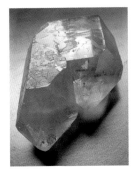

Rough twin crystal

Twin crystal:
two points from the same body.
Observe that there is no
division from the middle to
the base of the crystal.

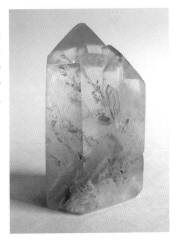

Citrine twin crystal

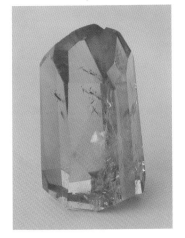

Rosy twin crystal

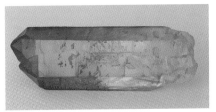

DOW CRYSTAL

The name of this quartz is a tribute to Jane Ann Dow, a great researcher of the metaphysical properties of crystals, and a friend of Katrina Raphael. However, this is not the only name by which this crystal is known; it is also referred to as 'trans-channelling' due to its capacity to transmit and channel energy and information.

A Dow crystal's point has six faces, three triangles alternating with three seven-sided faces.

- Manifestation of spiritual perfection in the material world: we can manifest the Divine (triangles) through contact with our inner truth (heptagons).

- Transmission of the Essence of Spirit into Earth's reality, that which can be seen, touched and understood.

- Contact with this crystal gradually brings about the under-standing that, in essence, everything exists in a state of perfection.
  - We can learn how to exist in the material world while maintaining the perfection of our spiritual essence.

Uses:
- For every situation that calls for the remembrance of this essence of 'perfection':
  - Conscious processes of mental and emotional re-program-ming.
  - Relationships.
  - Life issues that relate to judicial processes, professional performance, prosperity, etc.
  - To impregnate the aura, chakras, organs and cells with the essence of spiritual perfection, for health maintenance and to support a healing process.

DOW CRYSTAL

trans-channelling quartz crystal

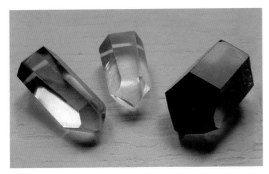

Citrine, clear, and smoky
Dow crystals

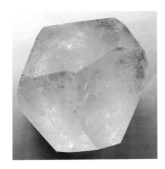

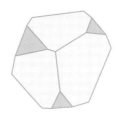

A perfect geometric pattern: 7:3:7:3:7:3.

Dow crystals with the phantom feature;
also known as Dow shaman

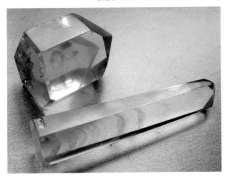

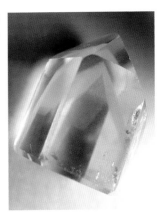

41

AGGREGATOR CRYSTAL

- Large crystal entirely or partially covered with smaller crystals.

- The large crystal is an 'old soul', containing wisdom and reliability that attracts the smaller crystals.

- The two main powers of this crystal are to attract and aggregate new or different:
  - Individuals
  - Ideas
  - Possibilities
  - Opportunities

- Pay attention to the meaning! To aggregate is not the same as to integrate, merge, unite or conciliate. 'To aggregate' implies 'to gather'.

- Useful when there are family, community or group problems.
  - Stimulates integration, cohesion and union in the group, as well as good will among group members.

- An excellent 'master' for people who are responsible for others and aggregate others, such as teachers, team leaders, and political or religious leaders.
  - Encourages responsibility, reliability, power, wisdom, love, compassion, resourcefulness and diplomacy.
  - Also balances group energy and relieves individual overburdening. Addresses the loss of individuality and privacy that can often occur with people who work as aggregators.

- Works with the energy of fertility, both physical and intellectual, encompassing the energies of prosperity and abundance.

AGGREGATOR CRYSTAL

 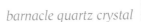
- Use a personal aggregator crystal to work with the concept of 'life experience':
  - We incarnate in order to have learning experiences.
  - We draft a script or a guide for our lives while in the spiritual world prior to incarnation.
  - We can use an aggregator crystal to attract and aggregate all types of resources and opportunities to facilitate our learning process in this incarnation.

Examples:

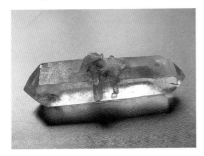 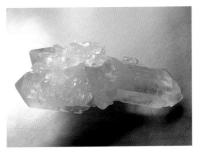

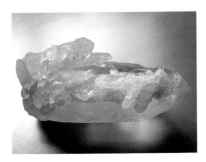 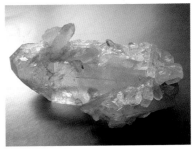

tabular quartz crystal

- Tabular quartzes have two opposite sides that are broader, giving them a flat body. They are usually double terminated, and in special cases are attached to other crystals in druses.

- Excellent aid for communication on all levels, both internally and externally:
  - Eliminates confusion, wrong interpretations and misunderstandings.
  - A major tool for communication with other realms.

- *The* channel for communication with the Higher Self.

- The power frequency of a tabular quartz is completely different from other quartz configurations. To this day its potential has not been duly acknowledged or utilized.

- A rare, powerful and potent crystal.

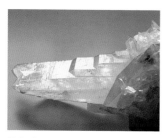

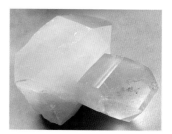

Tabular cathedral

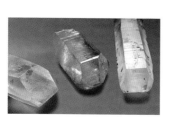

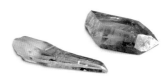

Tabular seed and double terminated tabular crystals

BRIDGE CRYSTAL

- A bridge crystal features at least one smaller crystal that penetrates the structure of the main crystal, and has part of its body inside the main crystal, and part outside.

- The smaller crystal(s) can penetrate into the larger crystal or project out from it.
  - We can consider the concept of 'a bridge going inside' and 'a bridge going outside'.

- Builds a bridge between the inner and outer worlds, myself and another, the inner child and the adult, the unconscious and conscious minds …

- The energy of a bridge crystal differs from the energy of the double terminated crystal. A bridge crystal *creates* an access, a path to allow communication and understanding. The double terminated crystal unblocks an existing access or path, and establishes communication through the energy of exchange and flow.

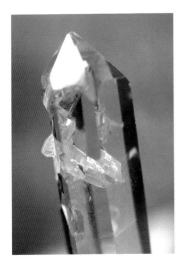
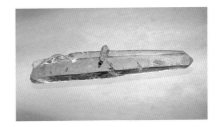
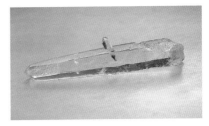

- The double terminated crystal captures and transmits energy through both its ends, and:

- Unites energies within its main body and then projects a new energy, the essence of which is a synthesis of the others - 'the great conciliator'.

- Dissolves stagnated energies.

- Promotes flow, movement.

- Balances.

- Integrates.

- Facilitates communication.

Some of the infinite possibilities for this crystal are to:

- Promote understanding, communication and idea exchange between two or more people.

- Balance the right and left hemispheres of the brain.

- Balance the yin/yang, masculine/feminine, electric/magnetic energies.

- Unblock energy accumulated in tissues, organs, chakras, or points within the body.

- Unblock the meridians, the vertical chain of force, and all the other paths our vital energy must follow in order to keep our bodies well fed and integrated.

- Promote a healing interchange by removing energy from an illness and replacing it with the energy of cure/balance.

DOUBLE TERMINATED CRYSTAL

double terminated quartz crystal

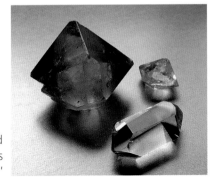

Naturally polished
double terminated crystals
resembling a 'balloon'

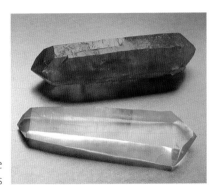

Double terminated tangerine
and clear quartz crystals

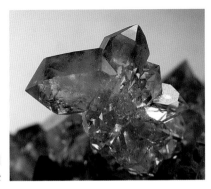

Detail of a double terminated
crystal druse

MANIFESTATION CRYSTAL

- A manifestation crystal is characterized as a larger crystal with a small crystal totally contained within it.

- Carries the knowledge of how we can manifest our dreams, desires and objectives in our material reality.

- Works with female fertility, and the ability to conceive and generate life.

- A symbol of the Divine Essence or Divine Spark within each of us.

Examples:

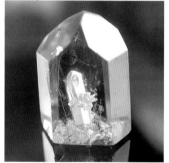 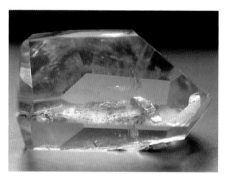

Some examples of manifestation crystals,
where a crystal has formed inside a bigger crystal.

SEED CRYSTAL

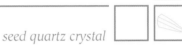

seed quartz crystal

- A seed crystal features a large base tapering to a point.

- Like the seed of a plant, a seed crystal contains the 'to be' energy, all the potential of what is to come.

- Uses:
    - To sow the seed of a new idea, a new beginning.
    - For New Year's rituals, to sow the seeds of wishes for the year ahead.
    - For a new business venture.
    - For the woman who wishes to become pregnant, so that the 'seed' may settle and germinate in the womb.
    - For male fertility.

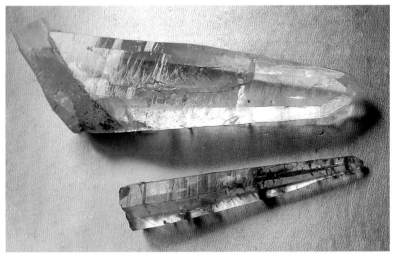

Examples of seed crystals in clear and citrine quartz.
Differs from a laser crystal in that it has a large base and tapers towards the point.

- Characterized by small crystalline structures formed in the region where the crystal was separated from its matrix.

- Despite having suffered damage during its growth or having been removed from its matrix, this crystal carries on its development to reach the state of perfection inherent in its nature, sometimes forming small, faceted terminations.

- Another type of self-healed crystal is one that has been broken and thus presents a visible fracture line.
  - The fracture is cured and the crystalline structure completed.

- Activates the self-healing and regenerating powers of our physical body, and also our power to overcome emotional issues such as the loss of a loved one, loss of a job, depression, etc.

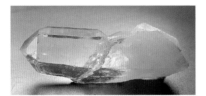
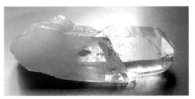

Self-healed crystal with a visible fracture line

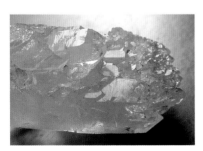
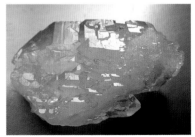

Self-healed crystal with faceted terminations

SCEPTRE CRYSTAL

sceptre quartz crystal

- The sceptres of kings and queens of all peoples have always symbolized superior power, the Divine Power, the legitimate power.

- The great teaching of this crystal: *only we have the power to create and change our own reality; everything begins and finishes within ourselves.*

- Helps us to learn how to integrate internal authority with external manifestation.

- Guides us towards who we really are, what we want, and how we can make manifest in the external world.

- Helps us to assume our role as creators.

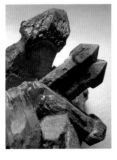

Power sceptres

A group of
power sceptres

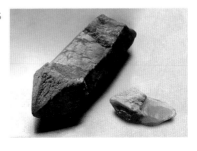

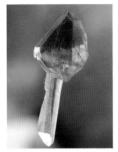

Double terminated power sceptres

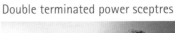

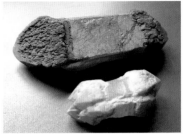

Power sceptre
with rutile

51

- Phantoms inside a crystal are indications of the crystal's evolutionary experiences and transformations.

- Phantom crystals had several lifetimes to learn how to be/exist in the same physical configuration.

- Represent the many stages of life we experience in a single incarnation.

- Symbolize universal wisdom.

- These are Earth stones to be used in the purification and redemption of our planet.
  - They work to unite people in taking action to save the planet.
  - Structures inside the crystal have a triangular-pyramidal formation, from which comes the energy to rescue, refresh and promote the spiritual healing of the Earth.

- Both the polished and the rough crystals are excellent energy sources for initiating a cure.

- Phantom crystals are excellent tools for meditation and to guide us in connecting to higher realms of wisdom.

- They carry knowledge that helps us to understand the reality of 'worlds inside worlds'; for example, the spiritual, mental, astral, etheric and physical planes.

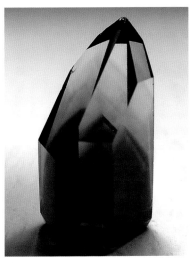

Citrine phantom

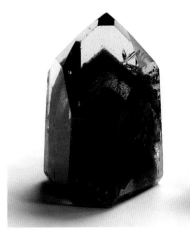

Black phantom

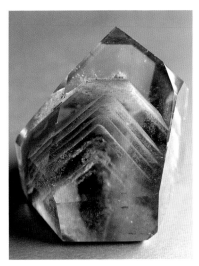

Phantom with inclusion

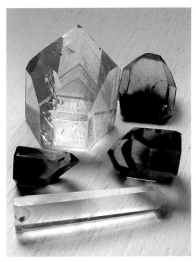

Diverse phantoms

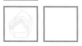
- Green phantom crystals are excellent carriers of healing energy and promote quick recovery/convalescence.

Examples:

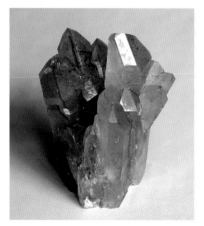

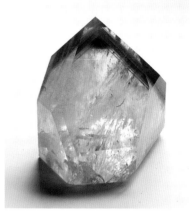

Green phantom cathedral

Example of green phantom crystals

Green phantom sphere

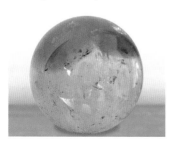

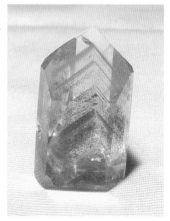

RAINBOW CRYSTAL

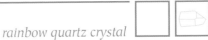
- Light expresses itself in infinite ways in the physical plane. Everything results from the play of light.

- A rainbow is the ultimate expression of light, representing all of creation.

- Quartzes have a remarkable ability to capture the rainbow. This is a very special gift from the guardian spirit of crystals.

- A rainbow crystal helps us to be multi-faceted in our own unique expression of light.

- Helps us to cope with negativity, while keeping in our consciousness the wisdom that love is at the basis of all life experiences.

- Possesses a deep and comprehensive healing energy because it contains all the primordial rays that gave birth to the cosmos.

- A wonderful tool to cure people from states of sadness, grief, or depression.

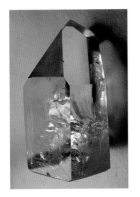
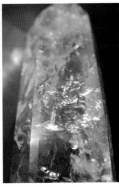
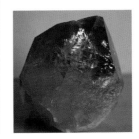

Various examples of rainbow crystals

A druse is characterised by two or more points or individualities growing from the same base. The individual crystals reflect light back and forth to one another, creating a powerful mantle in which all of them can bathe.

- The aura light of a druse is very strong.

- Each crystal (individuality) projects a specific energy, but each is related to the common base energy. Each works as a variation of one main theme.

- Each individual crystal points in a different direction, which makes the druse the most powerful instrument of energy diffusion and dissipation.

Druses and clusters symbolize civilizations or groups that have reached unity and harmony by satisfying the needs of each individual, while aligning personal goals with the needs of the whole.
'All for one and one for all!'

Base = Common purpose.

Each individual crystal = An aspect or person in a situation.

Druse/cluster = Everyone in harmonious cooperation, with respect for the individual, but aiming towards a common goal.

- Uses for a druse:

  1. To cleanse and energize:
     - Places
     - Other crystals
     - Objects: watches, jewelery, etc.

DRUSE

2. To disperse the unwanted energies of:
   - Microwaves, TVs, computers, mobile phones
   - Gutters, sewers, cesspits
   - Negative thoughts and feelings
   - Lower astral beings
   - Negative psychic interference

3. As an energy diffuser:
   - Acts as an amplifying and emitting base for the energies of other crystals.
   - Spreads the energies of harmony, cooperation, and respect for each person's individuality among the members of a company, family or other group.

4. In therapeutic settings:
   - For any part of the body that needs intensification of the energies of harmony and light.
   - Crystalline Harmonization Technique.

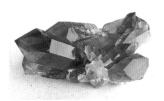

Smoky druse

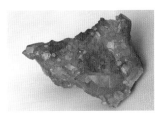

Tangerine druse

Rosy quartz druse

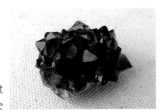

Amethyst druse

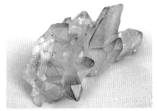

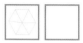

GENERATOR CRYSTAL

generator quartz crystal

- A generator crystal has a single termination, with six facets joining together to create the apex.

- Channels and grounds cosmic forces.

- Excellent for:
  - Meditation, to promote clarity and concentration.
  - Concentrating and distributing cosmic energy in strategic locations or in the centre of a mandala.
  - Creating a force field – can be used in every corner of a room, house or piece of land.
  - Cleansing and energizing the aura, chakras, or specific parts of the body.
  - Unblocking and activating the energy flow through the chakras and the acupuncture meridians.
  - Amplifying the healing energy of one's hands.

Example:

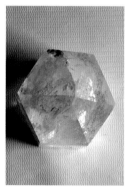 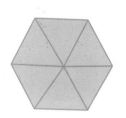 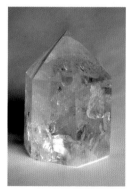

A crystal presenting a single termination, with six facets (triangles) joining together to create the apex.

ANCESTRAL CRYSTAL

ancestral quartz crystal

- An ancestral crystal presents marks resembling abrasions, sometimes likened to a bar code, in one or more sides and/or faces.

- The abrasions/marks are a code similar to hieroglyphs.

- These crystals contain information from Ancient Egypt, Lemuria, Atlantis, and other ancestral locations of the Universe.

- They were used in the healing temples of these civilizations and the abrasions contain information of the crystal's life experience, mainly relating to healing methods.

- The healing methods stored in an ancestral crystal can be understood and utilized in two ways:
  1. For our own healing and development.
  2. To help us help other people in their healing and development.

Examples:

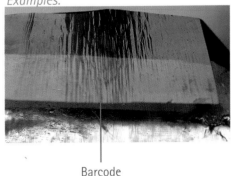

Barcode

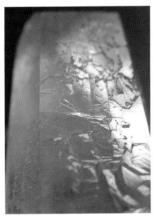

Abrasions

rutilated quartz crystal

- Rutiles are the most common minerals to be found as inclusions in the quartz family.

- Rutiles intensify the properties of the crystal in which they are included.

- A rutilated crystal is a very powerful accelerator because it generates and conveys electromagnetic energy that activates, accelerates and develops the issue that is being presented.

- Promote opening, growth and expansion.

- Eliminates any type of external interference and/or an eventual inner interference.

- Cleans and balances the aura as it repels dissonant energies.

- Perhaps the only crystal that can act upon the physical, etheric and emotional bodies.

- A rutilated crystal goes to the origin, the initial cause of a problem:
  - Like a programmed missile, it scans our being, inside and out, until it finds the core of the problem.
  - The rutile needles 'explode' the condensed/crystallized nucleus of the energy that is causing the problem, emptying it.
  - From this point, therapies and solutions can start to perform freely and have their effects accelerated.

- Amplifies our powers of creation and manifestation.

- Rutiles can be found seperately in nature.

- Colours of rutiles known to this date: red, copper, gold, silver, black, blue, yellow, white, green, pink and violet.

RUTILATED CRYSTAL

rutilated quartz crystal

Caution:
Because a rutilated crystal is a powerful producer and conductor of electromagnetic energy, its continuous use in jewellery must be cautioned as it can cause agitation, anxiety, tachycardia, headaches and nausea, and can increase the predisposition for static shocks from car doors, fridges, etc.

Examples:

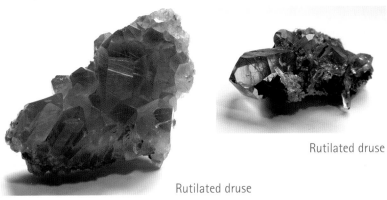

Rutilated druse

Rutilated druse

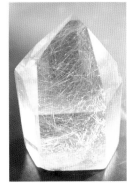
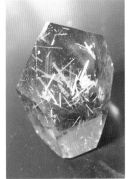
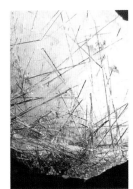

RECORD KEEPER CRYSTAL

- A record keeper crystal has one or more triangles visible on one or more of its faces.

- A record keeper crystal can record aeons of wisdom and reveal ancient knowledge and deep secrets of the Universe.
  - Each triangle recorded on the crystal is an eye of the crystal, and a portal to powerful wisdom.

- A record keeper crystal contains information about the soul of the human race and about everything that exists in this reality.

- They were programmed in an intentional and conscious way by the beings that created the conditions that made possible the evolution of human life on Earth, or by their successors in Lemuria and Atlantis.
  - These evolved beings came from far beyond the solar system and arrived on Earth to give origin to the first race.
  - They wanted to preserve the secrets of the Universe so that the human soul, once ready, would be able to inherit the wisdom of the cosmos.
  - These crystals were specially chosen to be programmed with galaxies of information, and then buried in the womb of the Earth so that they would come to the surface only at the appropriate time, to be used by the right people.

- Record keepers 'come' to us. Often a crystal goes from hand to hand, and then suddenly the triangle manifests itself when it is in contact with a certain person.

- A record keeper crystal promotes the actualization of each individual as an agent of healing.

- Record keeper crystals help to bring superior knowledge, wisdom, peace and love to this and other planets.

record keeper quartz crystal

- Handling a record keeper crystal is a big responsibility.
  - Information received can differ from everything that has been seen or experienced before.
  - There can be data that doesn't relate at all with physical life on this planet.
  - The receiver needs to train his/her mind to be open to inconceivable concepts, and be able to process them somehow in his/her life.
  - The purpose of receiving all this extraordinary information is not to escape from the terrestrial world, but rather to incorporate higher wisdom, love and peace into our Earthly existence.

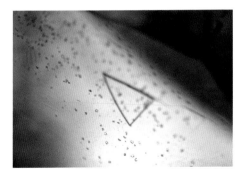

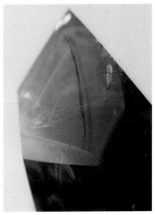

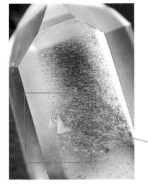

Detail: Emphasis on the triangles for improved visibility.

Examples of record keeper crystals.

TRIGONIC CRYSTAL

- A trigonic crystal is a quartz crystal with small triangles pointing upward, towards the termination of the crystal, and downward, towards the base of the crystal.

- The triangles are naturally chiselled and embossed.

- A Brazilian crystal, and very rare nowadays.

- This crystal became 'famous' when Jane Ann Dow (who, along with Katrina Raphael, was a pioneer in bringing forward the metaphysical knowledge of crystals) began using it to work with terminally ill patients.

- An initiation crystal (maybe the only one).

- Provides access to superconsciousness: the 'chain' of triangles is the link between our consciousness and superconsciousness.

- Teaches us that we need to understand ourselves and all of creation from a spiritual perspective.
  - Each triangle is a key to wisdom we may acquire in this and other lives.

- Uses:
  - When we are called to begin our soul's journey.
  - To solidify new patterns of consciousness.
  - In the death process (upwards triangles) – transition from matter to spirit.
  - During pregnancy, delivery, and the baby's first three months of life (downwards triangles) – to welcome someone new to the world.

TRIGONIC CRYSTAL

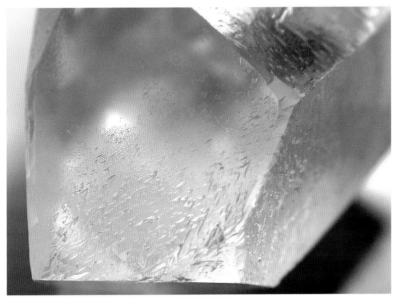

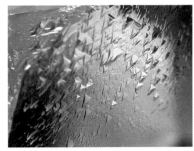 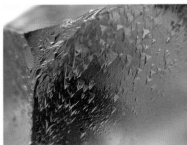

Examples of trigonic crystals: surface marked by 'triangles'.

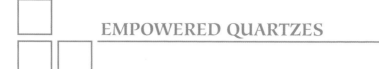

The forms I have described in this chapter manifest in different types of quartz – amethyst, citrine, clear, smoky, tangerine and rosy quartz – that may also contain rutiles.

There are also some examples where two or more special forms may be present. I call these 'empowered quartzes'.

It is important to explore the different characteristics of a crystal in order to obtain the best result when it is used. I will be offering some examples, but an interpretation is always very personal, and also reflects only the present moment in your life. Each person will place emphasis on different properties – on a special form (a window crystal for instance), on constitution (possibly a druse or double terminated quartz), or on the type of quartz (clear, amethyst, tangerine, etc.).

Example – The presence of an Isis form:

a) In the end of a smoky quartz – The energy of the Goddess is anchored in the physical plane (smoky quartz). We can use it to help us dissolve blockages and negativity that prevent the manifestation of this energy in our lives, and to build the structure necessary to integrate this aspect into our lives.

b) In the end of a rutilated smoky quartz – The properties of the smoky quartz are intensified, making it suitable for cases where the blockages and negativities are denser and/or there is a need to accelerate the process of retrieving and integrating the energy of the Goddess in the physical plane.

c) In a clear quartz druse – Could be used to help a group of people or a family that is receiving the gifts of the Goddess: perseverance, determination, the power to overcome.

d) In one of the extremities of a double-terminated clear quartz – Could be used to establish a relationship, a compliance or an exchange between your energy and the energy of the Goddess.

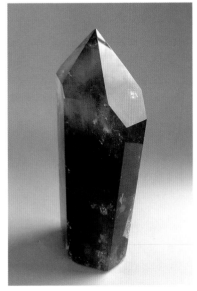

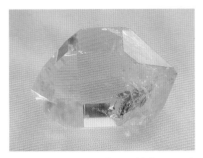

Double terminated Isis crystal

Smoky Isis crystal

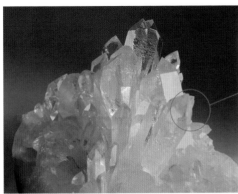

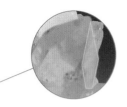

Druse with Isis

Now let us imagine an even more complex example: a clear quartz druse that presents an Isis *and* a window configuration.

We are in the presence of a very special and powerful crystal. How can we interpret so many different energies in a single crystal?

One of the possible interpretations: This is a crystal to help a group of people (druse) that are joined together (perhaps all members of a study group) to seek within their essence or Self (window crystal) the presence of the Goddess or the feminine aspect of God (Isis crystal).

Examples:

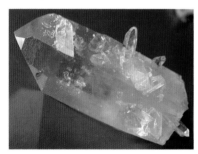

Clear quartz: aggregator, bridge, rainbow, self-healed

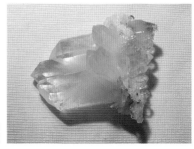

Clear quartz: cathedral, bridge, double terminated

MY
PERSONAL
EXPERIENCE

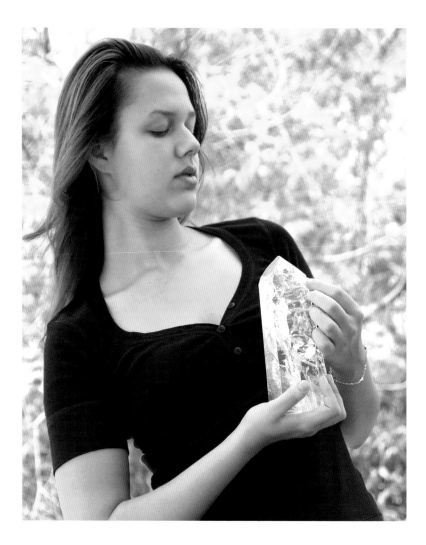

Crystals are extremely powerful instruments for connecting with ourselves and with the Universe. Remember, however, that the greatest power is inside you.

Do not transfer your power to anybody or any thing! Work with your heart, your intuition, your feelings, and with your imagination!

MY PERSONAL EXPERIENCE

Dear reader, now I want to share how I use the energies of crystals in my daily life. I will remind you again that there are neither prescriptions nor any absolute truths when it comes to crystals.

Relationships with crystals are personal because crystals 'speak' to our souls. This is why I have learned to give credit and respect to every person's point of view and intuition.

The crystals I have at home most often are druses, especially clear quartz and amethyst, because they have the power to disperse negative/stagnant energies, and to diffuse the positive energies of light and harmony.

AMETHYST DRUSES

Amethyst is a representative of the mineral kingdom that condenses and embodies the seventh ray (violet ray). Its properties are: liberation, transformation, transmutation, protection, mercy and compassion.

How I use them:

a) In bathrooms
- Location: A druse of approximately 10 cm, kept as close as possible to the toilet seat.
- Intention: To transform and transmute 'ending, excrement energies'.

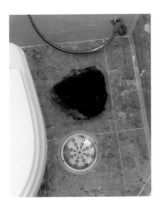

b) In bedrooms
- Location: A druse of approximately 10 cm, kept at the bedside (near the head), on the floor or on the bedside table.
- For double beds, one on each bedside.
- Intention: A good night's sleep.

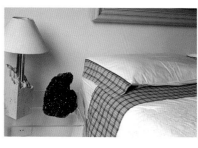

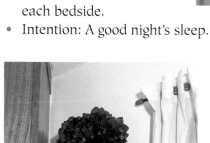

- Location: A larger druse of a minimum of 10 cm, located, if possible, in a high position, for instance on a high shelf, or in a corner opposite the bed.
- Intention: Keep protection and energy levels high whilst we sleep.

c) In the living room
In this part of the house I also have a large clear quartz druse of 20-50 cm, placed in a strategic spot, my intention being to encourage the energy of harmonious companionship among two or more people while respecting each one's individuality.

d) Other critical spots

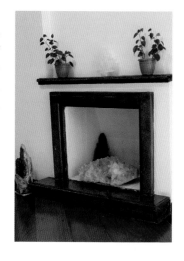

1. Computer/TV
- Location: A clear or amethyst druse of approximately 10 cm, close to the monitor /screen.
- Intention: Disperse, transform, and transmute harmful electromagnetic energies, and spread positive energies.

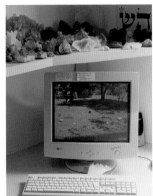

2. Microwave oven
- Location: a clear quartz or amethyst druse of approximately 10 cm on top of the microwave or as close as possible to it.
- Intention: Disperse, transform, and transmute harmful electromagnetic energies and spread positive energies.

A CRYSTALLINE ALTAR

As you can imagine, I have many crystals.

Through the study of shamanism I learned to set up an altar, a special place where I put everything that is sacred to me, everything that brings me a feeling of reverence for our Creator, for creation, and for Life. I have transferred this knowledge to the creation of a crystalline altar.

In the stand where my crystals are displayed, I reserve a space where I keep my personal crystals. These are the crystals that touch me deeply and they are only used by me. I also place in this reserved space the crystals I am currently working with. At the top of the altar, as if it were a pointer, I place a cathedral quartz with the intention of marking this area as my Sacred Space, and around the cathedral I arrange the other crystals.

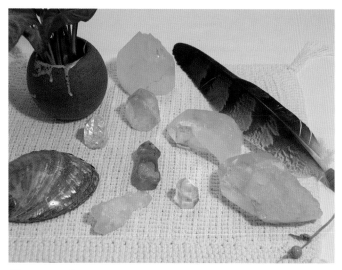

Altar example

Some examples:

- Isis quartz symbolizing my relation with the Goddess energy.
- Tabular quartz, which is also self-healed, symbolizing recovering and learning with my Self or Higher Self.
- Self-healed quartz, symbolizing the activation of my self healing, regeneration and my power to overcome.
- Window quartz, the mirror of my soul.
- Power sceptre quartz, symbolizing my process of learning to understand, accept and exercise my power to create and manifest my own reality.
- Clear Dow phantom quartz, to symbolize and remind me that perfection is inherent in everything that is manifested, including myself.
- Aggregator quartz, which is also a bridge, double terminated crystal, specially chosen to help me exercise my position as an 'opinion shaper', in the correct way, through my courses and lectures.

With this arrangement I have many intentions:

- May the Universe bring me all the necessary external and internal resources so that I may transmit 'mineral kingdom medicine' in a sacred manner.
- May I have the wisdom to be in constant balance between responsibility and overload; in other words, to recognise whether I am helping someone or 'carrying' them.

GROUPING WITH SPECIFIC AIMS

I group and display some crystals in a particular way in order to activate the main areas of my life:

Love and Relationship
Next to a picture of my partner and me:

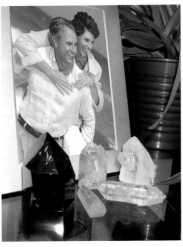

- Twin quartz to help the process of learning inside a true and deep relationship, a relationship between souls.
- Double terminated quartz to improve communication and energy exchange.
- Bridge quartz so that a bridge may link our bodies, hearts, minds and souls.
- Self-healed quartz to help our capacity for constant re-construction, regeneration, recreation and renewal in our relationship.
- Smoky quartz to help us build a solid and structured relation-ship.

Prosperity
- many, many citrines.
- Tangerine double terminated quartz: to guarantee a free and continuous flow between me and prosperity.
- Tangerine quartz druse: prosperity for all.

Protection
- Smoky quartz.
- Rutilated crystals, in particular with black rutiles.
- Laser crystals facing outwards, in a semicircle around crystals mentioned above, to create an 'invisibility field'.

You can also arrange groups of crystals with specific purposes for another person, or for a situation you wish to work on.

For a person, put his/her picture in the centre, or write his/her full name and date of birth on unlined paper and place it in the centre.

For a specific situation, place something in the centre that represents the situation, such as a picture, a letter, an advertisement, etc. You can also describe the situation on a piece of paper (this time it does not need to be without lines).

To select crystals to be used, always use your intuition.

Perhaps the following suggestion can help you in the beginning:
- Assemble all the crystals that you feel would serve your purpose.
- Sit comfortably in front of them and close your eyes.
- Breathe deeply as many times as needed to relax and clear your mind.
- Still with your eyes closed, concentrate and visualize the person or problem, and your purpose. Do not hurry; immerse yourself in the vision.

- When you feel ready, open your eyes slowly and contemplate the crystals, without expectation or anxiety.
- You will feel the need or impulse to take one or more crystal(s) in your hands. Do so.
- Continue to contemplate the crystals until you feel you have chosen all those needed for your work.
- Assemble the chosen crystals in way that feels meaningful to you, in a separate place.
- Energize the arrangement in a way that feels suitable to you (through prayer, Reiki, etc.), but most of all visualize the light from the crystals involving and penetrating the person or situation.
- Contemplate the arrangement from time to time.

CLEANSING A CRYSTAL ARRANGEMENT

- Rearrange the crystals if you feel the need; feel free to remove or add a new crystal.
- Energize the assembly once again if you have made a rearrangement.
- When you feel that your objective has received the necessary light, dismantle the arrangement.
- Wash the crystals under running water and leave them in the open air for one or more days, or for however long you feel this process requires.

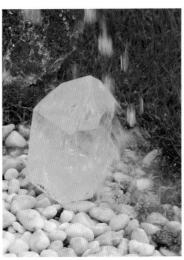

FINAL CONSIDERATIONS

Dear reader,

I would like to mention again some important points:

- Crystals are only instuments, powerful of course, but only instruments.
  - As is the case with any tool, they are not essential. However, they do make things easier.
  - After working for a while with your crystals, if you discover that you can do without them with efficiency and effectiveness... great! Leave them on display so that you can continue to contemplate their beauty, and just carry on with your work.

- There is no right or wrong, no absolute truth in any field of knowledge, least of all in relation to crystals.
  - Above all else, try to be loyal to your intuition: when you feel a strong impulse or a clear indication to choose a crystal, this is much more valuable than information acquired from a book or a lecture. Even if your intuitions contradict all the 'rules'.

- If we truly believe and it makes deep sense to us, then it will work.

- We can and should each create our own methods for using crystals.

BIBLIOGRAPHY

Bravo, Brett – *O segredo dos cristais – Um Guia Prático*, São Paulo, Editora Pensamento, 1997

Cavalcanti, Virgínia – *Cristal não é aspirina*, São Paulo, Editora Objetiva, 1993

Cunningham, Scott – *Crystals Encyclopedia, precious stones and metals*, São Paulo, Editora Gaia, 2005

Duncan, Antônio, *O Caminho das Pedras*, Rio de Janeiro, Editora Nórdica, 1998

Melody, *Love is in the Earth, a Kaleidoscope of Crystals – Updated*, Colorado, Earth-Love Publishing House, 2004

Raphael, Katrina, *A Cura pelos Cristais*, São Paulo, Editora Pensamento, 2005

Raphael, Katrina, *Transmissões Cristalinas*, São Paulo, Editora Pensamento, 1992

Raphael, Katrina – *As Propriedades Curativas dos Cristais e das Pedras Preciosas*, São Paulo, Editora Pensamento, 2005

Crystal lectures course material by Claudine Camas.

All the important information about 430 healing gemstones in a neat pocket book! Michael Gienger, known for his popular introductory work *Crystal Power, Crystal Healing,* here presents a comprehensive directory of all the gemstones currently in use. In a clear, concise and precise style, with pictures accompanying the text, the author describes the characteristics and healing functions of each crystal.

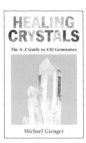

Michael Gienger
Healing Crystals
The A - Z Guide to 430 Gemstones
Paperback, 96 pages
ISBN 978-1-84409-067-9

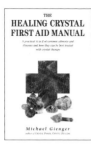

This is an easy-to-use A-Z guide for treating many common ailments and illnesses with the help of crystal therapy. It includes a comprehensive colour appendix with photographs and short descriptions of each gemstone recommended.

Michael Gienger
The Healing Crystals First Aid Manual
A Practical A to Z of Common Ailments and Illnesses and How They Can Be Best Treated with Crystal Therapy
288 pages, with 16 colour plates
ISBN 978-1-84409-084-6

For further information and book catalogue contact:
Findhorn Press, 305a The Park, Forres IV36 3TE, Scotland.
Earthdancer Books is an Imprint of Findhorn Press.

tel +44 (0)1309-690582   fax +44 (0)1309-690036

info@findhornpress.com   www.findhornpress.com   www.earthdancer.co.uk

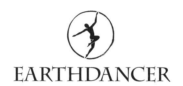

EARTHDANCER

A FINDHORN PRESS IMPRINT